Disclaimer Notice:

Please note the information contained within this document is for education and entertainment purpose only. All effort has been executed to present accurate, up to date, reliable, complete information. No warranties of any kind are declared or implied. Readers acknowledge that the author is not engaged in the rendering of legal, financial, medical or professional advice. The content within this book has been derived from various sources. Please consult a licensed professional before attempting any techniques outlined in this book.

Contents

Introduction 5

Chapter One 6

Chapter Two..8

    Best Practises and Filter to Use 8

    Is it possible to stop germs, bacteria and virus while

    using a face mask? 8

    What type of filter is possible to use? 9

Chapter Three...11

    Super Practical Homemade Mask.................................. 11

    The Required Material 11

    The Steps To Follow: 12

Chapter Four 16

    Sew Your Protective Mask in Washable Fabric............. 16

    Materials For One Fabric Mask:.............................. 16

    Matching Sewing Thread 16

Chapter Five 19

    Create a Fabric Face Mask 19

Introduction

The surgical face mask has become the symbol of the epidemic, the ultimate tool to avoid contamination, and everyone wants their own. Since the start of the coronavirus epidemic, surgical masks have been torn off, and hospitals fear the shortage of this tool necessary for the protection of nursing staff. This object is the subject of a daily battle between the government and the citizens, in order to avoid the shortage. An alternative method is the homemade protective face mask.

These homemade versions are now available on prescription. They, therefore, do not aim to cure Covid-19 but to avoid contamination of others when one is carrying the virus. As a reminder, the absence of symptoms does not mean that you are healthy: it is therefore recommended to wear a mask when you are brought into contact with other people. If the effectiveness of these homemade face masks is not proven and is the subject of many debates, many consider them as a first barrier against the virus, avoiding the projection of droplets or the contact of his hand with his mouth after touching a potentially contaminated surface. In addition, sewing a protective mask preserves the stocks of approved surgical masks - already very limited. We also think of cashiers, police and gendarmes, driver. Making a homemade mask for all these people can, therefore, help protect them and protect us at the same time.

Today we have time for once—time to do what we never take the time to do. Take advantage of his own. Focus on essential things. But also make yourself useful and help each other. A call for help has been issued; we are out of protective face masks to protect ourselves from the Coronavirus and prevent its spread. A 100% do it yourself face mask, which, in addition to offering a minimum means of protection, allows time to pass during this period of confinement.

Chapter One

You may have heard a lot recently about using face masks to prevent infection. One recent study found that Google searches related to face masks have spiked up. So, are face masks effective, and if so, when should you wear them and what type should you use?

What Are The Two Primary Types Of Face Masks?

When you hear about face masks for COVID-19 prevention, it's generally two types:

1. The surgical mask
2. The N95 respirator

Let's explore each of them in a little more detail below.

- **Surgical masks**

these are designed to catch your bodily fluids such as saliva and nasal discharge, thus preventing the infectious liquid droplets from spreading to other people.

- **N95 respirators**

An N95 respirator is a more tight-fitting face mask. In addition to splashes, sprays, and large droplets, this respirator can also filter out 95 percent of microscopic particles. This includes viruses and bacteria. It is the most effective in fighting the virus.

When And How To Wear Face Mask Due To Virus

Disposable face masks can only be used once. The WHO notes that if you are not ill or taking care of a patient, you are wasting a mask, worsening the current global shortage.

How Do You Remove And Dispose Of A Face Mask?

To remove the mask, remove it from behind (do not touch the front of the mask); discard immediately in a closed bin. Face mask becomes a hazard for others if carelessly disposed of. If you wear a mask, then you must know how to use it and dispose of it properly. Perform hand hygiene after touching or discarding the mask. Use alcohol-based hand rub or, if visibly soiled, wash your hands with soap and water.

Chapter Two

Best Practises and Filter to Use

We have seen what is and how to correctly use a face mask, it could be useful to understand what are the best practices to adopt while using a protective face mask and what kind of filters are useful.

Is it possible to stop germs, bacteria and virus while using a face mask?

A lot of factors influence the spread of viruses and bacteria despite the use of protective face mask. We need to pay attention to the type of face mask we are using, the way it is used, how long it is used, the place in which the individual stay, etc. Furthermore, we cannot say that the face mask itself prevent totally from becoming sick, but to answer properly to this question it is better to understand how someone could be infected when they come in contact with a sick person. Viruses and bacteria spread out in many ways, but, if a person is infected, the disease could be transmitted via *airborne respiratory droplets*, or by dir*ect contact with nasal and throat secretions*. If this sick individual coughs or sneezes or touch the eyes and nose and then touch another person or a surface, the someone who come into contact with these contagious droplets - either in the air or by touching a surface that contained the droplets - this person, too, could get sick.

Because of this, the most basic and efficient way to limit or even stop the spread in a country of contagious disease, is to **impose a lockdown to the infected area** and, consequently, a quarantine to all the individuals of this area, either they are sick yet or not.

The second basic rule of thumb that can both help us and limit the contagion, is **wearing a face mask and washing constantly our hands**. Two studies reinforced this concept:

one from 2008 found that less than 20% of those who used a mask were likely to get the flu, another carried out in 2009, found that face masks and frequent hand-washing lowered people's risk of getting the flu by about 70%.

Stated that, it is important not to get confused. *If only wearing a face mask is helpful but not at all because it still leave the eyes open so that they can be touch by the sick person, the second important fact to notice is that wearing a face mask is the best thing a sick person can do to protect the other people! In fact, if we consider the **severe acute respiratory syndrome (SARS)** epidemic that happened in 2003, the researchers discovered that the main role that face masks played, especially in the hospitals, has been mostly essential to prevented sick people from passing SARS around, to protect others from harmful viruses and germs.*

What type of filter is possible to use?

A filter is a material that obstacle particles from passing through by capturing them. Obviously, the less particles pass through and, together, the smallest the particles that are blocked are, the more efficient the material used as a filter is. Therefore, what are the best materials commercially available to be used as filter?

The most common materials that can be used are:

- **Silk**
- **Linen**
- **Pillowcase**
- **Scarf**
- **Cotton**
- **Dish Towel**

A study of the Cambridge University (*Testing the Efficacy of Homemade Masks: Would They Protect in an Influenza Pandemic?* [1]) tested all of these materials to capture **0.02**

micron Bacteriophage MS2 particles (5 times smaller than the coronavirus) and stated them in a scale from *the worst, the Scarf*, which shown itself to <u>be able to block the 49%</u> of these very small particles, to *the better, the Dish Towel and the Cotton Blend* (material of a common T-shirt) that are <u>successful in capturing the 70% of particles</u>.

So the most common materials available at home are efficient enough to be used as filter, if we double it the percentage of blockage increase dramatically, but before cutting out mask from all the Dish Towels that are at home, is is important to consider also the *breathability* of such materials. Still this study concludes saying that *"The pillowcase and the 100% cotton t-shirt were found to be the most suitable household materials for an improvised face mask"*.

---

[1]https://www.researchgate.net/publication/258525804_Testing_the_Efficacy_of_Homemade_Masks_Would_They_Protect_in_an_Influenza_Pandemic

Here after it is shown a further material, MERV-13, which is possible to buy and that could be best solution as filter.

Chapter Three

Super Practical Homemade Mask

To make an effective homemade mask, it is necessary to synthesize between a well-adjusted pattern, a quality fabric, and several layers of suitable fabric.

Rendering of the mask

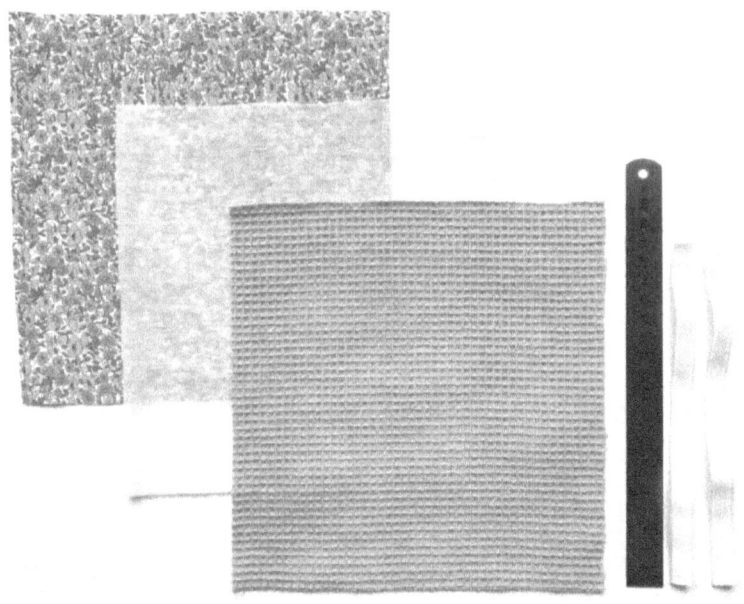

The Required Material

- ☐ Two 20x20 cm squares of fabric

- ☐ 1 square the same size as a fusible, and

- ☐ Two 18 cm elastic bands

- ☐ Filter

You can get all the materials at Amazon or Alibaba website.

The Steps To Follow:

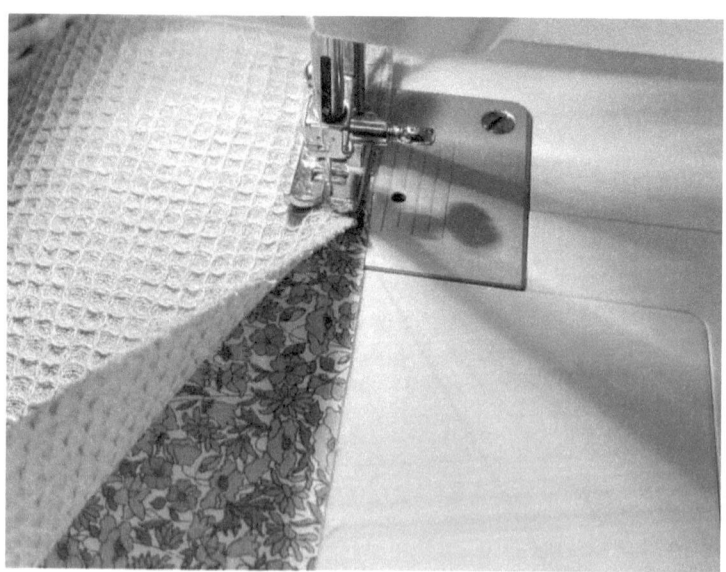

- **Sew right sides together**

Sew two parallel edges which will become the top and bottom

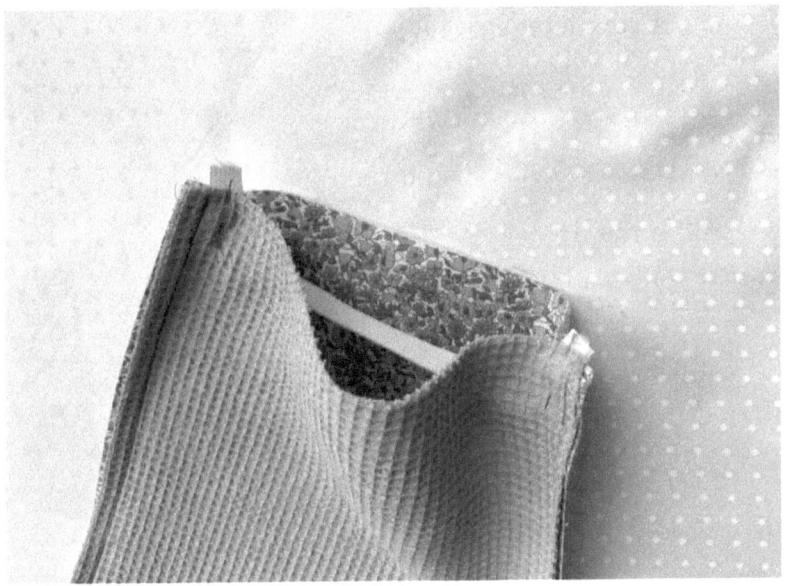

- **Arrange the elastics**

On each side, place the elastic bands in the corners, forming a loop.

And put your filter as well

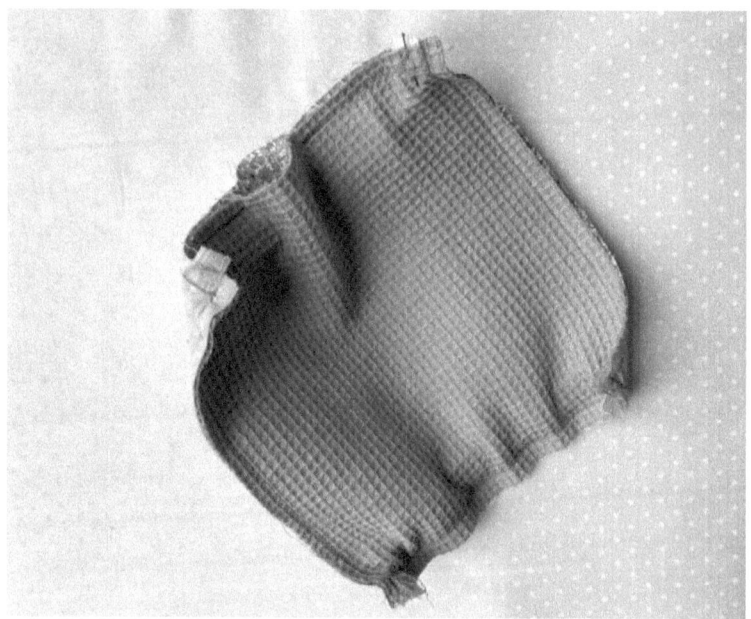

- **Sew with a slit**

Sew both sides, leaving an open slit 6 cm.

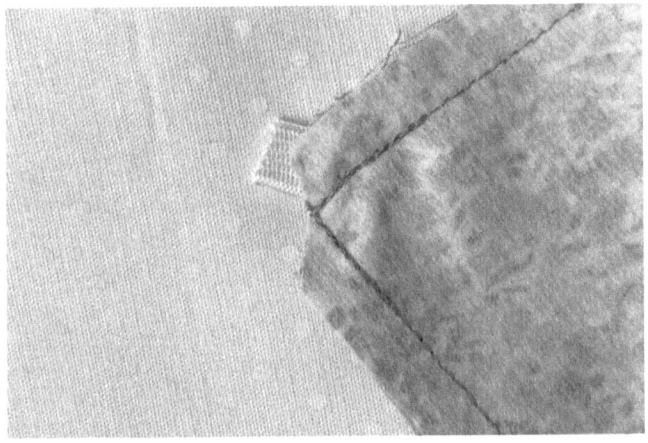

- **Notching the angles**

Take care not to damage the elastic

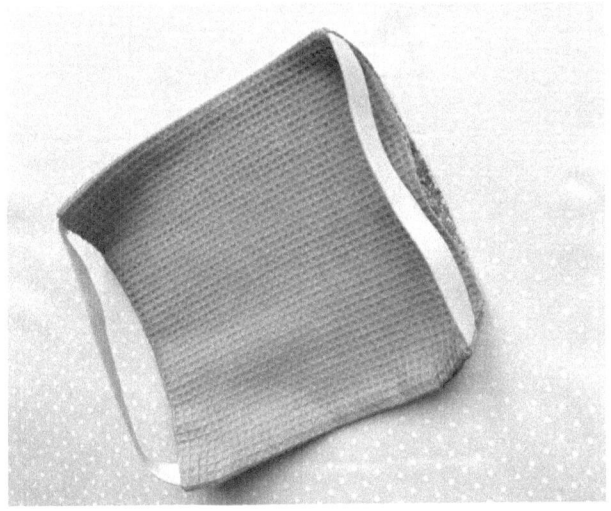

- **Turn over, close the slot and iron**

Carefully iron the resulting square

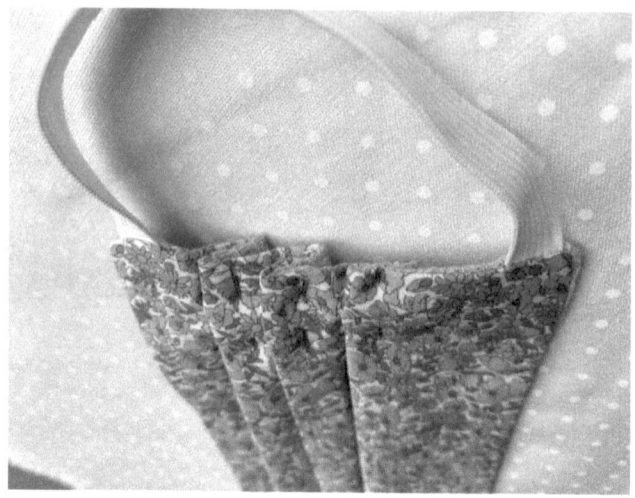

- **Form the folds**

Form 3 folds of 1 cm accordion.

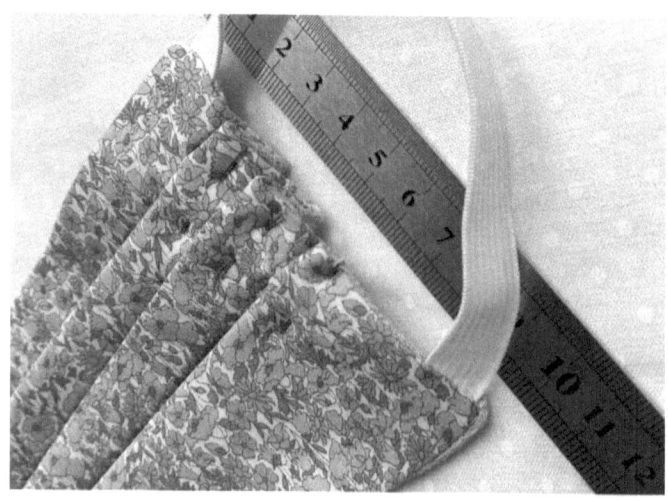

- **Iron these folds carefully**

The height must be 10 cm in total

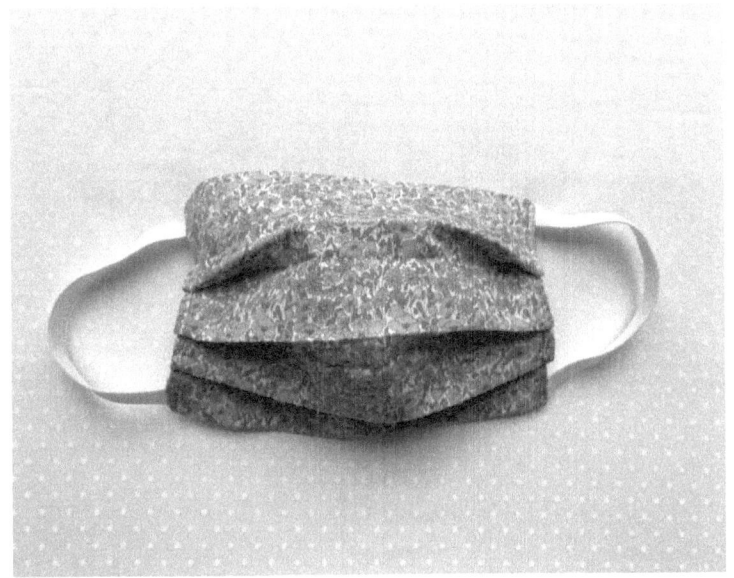

- **Sew the folds as close as possible to the edges**

Sew, taking care that the folds remain parallel to the top and bottom sides.

Chapter Four

Sew Your Protective Mask in Washable Fabric

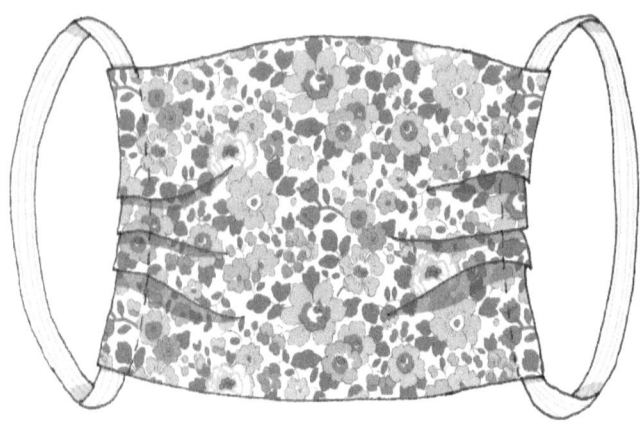

Materials For One Fabric Mask:

1. Outer fabric: 21 X 19 cm (adult), 19 X 17 cm (child)

2. Lining: 21 X 19 cm (adult), 19 X 17 cm (child)

You can get all the materials at Amazon or Alibaba website.

Matching Sewing Thread

It is advisable to choose fine to medium fabrics and to double the layers of fabrics to have four layers of fabric or to insert a layer of <u>fine fleece</u> or <u>fleece</u> (100% polyester).

1. According to the pattern, cut a rectangle in the outer fabric and a rectangle in the lining. Mark the marks for the folds. Pin the pleats at the marks and build them to maintain them.

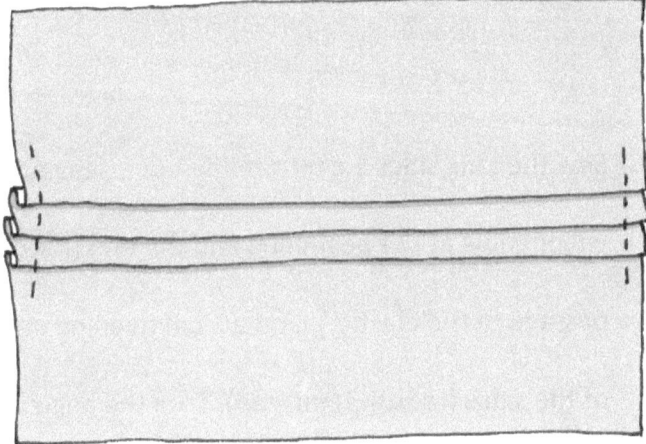

2. Place the two rectangles right sides together (marking the folds well). Sew the short sides 1 cm from the edge, starting and stopping the seam 1 cm from the ends.

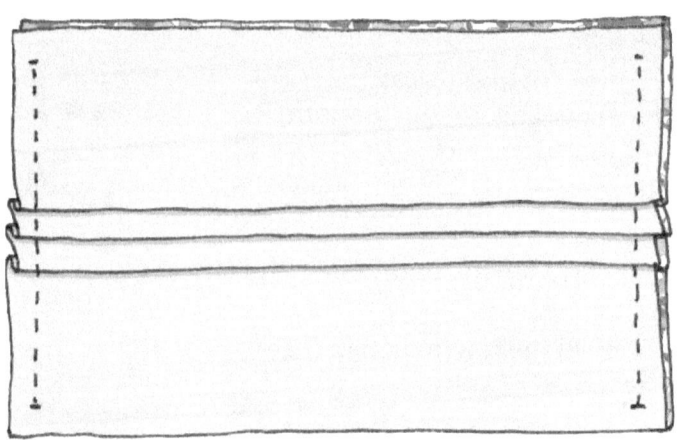

3. Sew the long sides 1 cm from the edge, leaving a 1 cm opening at the beginning and the end (for the passage of the elastics), and a 5 cm opening on one of the sides (to turn right side). Trim the angles.

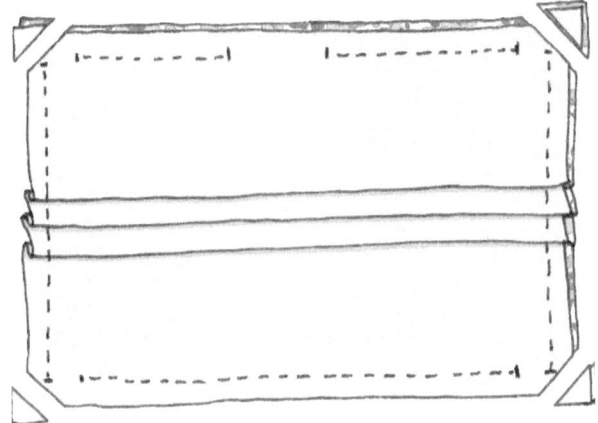

4. Return to the right side, then close the invisible stitch opening. Topstitch the short sides 1 cm from the edge, then slide the elastic with a safety pin. Sew the end of the elastics securely.

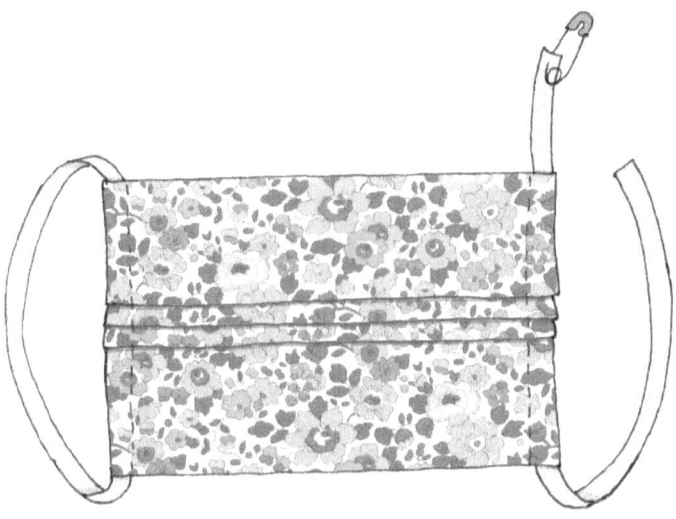

Chapter Five

Create a Fabric Face Mask

Because of the shortage of oral masks, Public Health advises all responsible citizens to make their mask in order to leave professional masks to medical services, medical staff, hospitals, doctors, nurses, and other professionals. Here is another way to make yours.

Materials:

1. 2 squares of fabric of 20 x 20 cm (here we used thick cotton and a honeycomb)

2. One iron-on patch of 20 x 20 cm

3. Filter

4. Two elastic bands of 18 cm each or two fine strips of cloth

You can get all the materials at Amazon or Alibaba website.

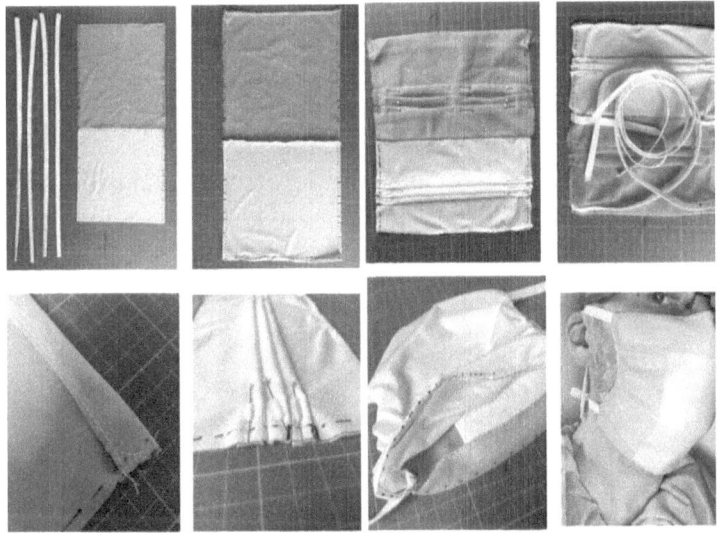

The Steps To Make A Fabric Mask:

1. Paste one of the two fabrics to solidify it and to "seal it" further.

2. Pin, right sides together, the two squares of material (including the one that has been heating sealed). Stitch on two opposite sides which will become the top and the bottom.

3. Slide the ends of an elastic band or the fine strip of cloth into each corner and pin it by forming a loop inside the mask. Sew. Do the same on the opposite

edge, making sure to leave a 6 cm slit so that you can turn the mask over.

4. Place your filter, iron and notch the angles, taking care not to cut the elastics.

5. Turn over and bring out the edges with a pen tip. Iron. Close the slit by sewing by hand with slip stitches.

6. Form three flat folds in the middle of the mask: fold the fabric over 1 cm (well parallel to the top and bottom) and by folding this fold down. Repeat twice. Iron.

7. Stitch these folds as close as possible to the edge. It's over!

Chapter Six

Using MERV 13 Air Filter to Improve the Performance of Your Mask

What is **MERV 13 Air Filter** and why it is useful? Before going deeper and explaining how it is possible to use such a filter to create a better face mask, it is important to state few but important concepts that can help to understand why this "recipe" can develop the best in performance face mask that everyone can create at home.

Indoor air pollution is an ongoing study that brought to the concept of **Indoor Air Quality** (**IAQ**), a research that have established that there are many little slivers of invisible pieces that float around in the air. Those particulates, or **particulate matter** (**PM 2.5**, everything that is 2.5 micrometres or smaller) can penetrate deeper into the lungs and from here even into the blood. This can easily lead to respiratory disease, especially which that are related to indoor air pollution.

For this reason, it has been studied a wide range of materials that can be used to create air filter. Furthermore, it has been developed and adopted a new measurement scale, formed by 16 rating levels, that "represents a quantum leap in the precision and accuracy of air-cleaner ratings": *Minimum Efficiency Reporting Value*, abbreviated MERV. Each level is related to the percentage efficacy of the air filter to block the particles from passing through.

The *MERV 13* is the minimum level that allows to retain PM in the range from 1.0 to 0.3 micrometres, the rage considered adapt to stop bacteria and that is therefore used in hospitals and general surgery applications. In conclusion, using a MERV 13 air filter is the best way possible to strengthen our face mask.

Materials:

1. 2 squares of fabric of 20 x 20 cm (here we used thick cotton and a honeycomb)

2. One iron-on patch of 20 x 20 cm

3. One MERV-12 Air Filter

4. Two elastic bands of 18 cm each or two fine strips of cloth

You can get all the materials at Amazon or Alibaba website.

The steps are similar to what has been explained in the chapter before, the only new information is regarding how to use and involve the filter in the procedure.

The Steps To Make A MERV-13 Filter Face Mask:

1. An air filter of this kind is easy to find on Amazon or Alibaba, but before sewing the mask is important

to know how to use it. The filter is placed in a frame, so we need to carefully strip it down and obtain only the layer. Here below an example of how this filter could looks like.

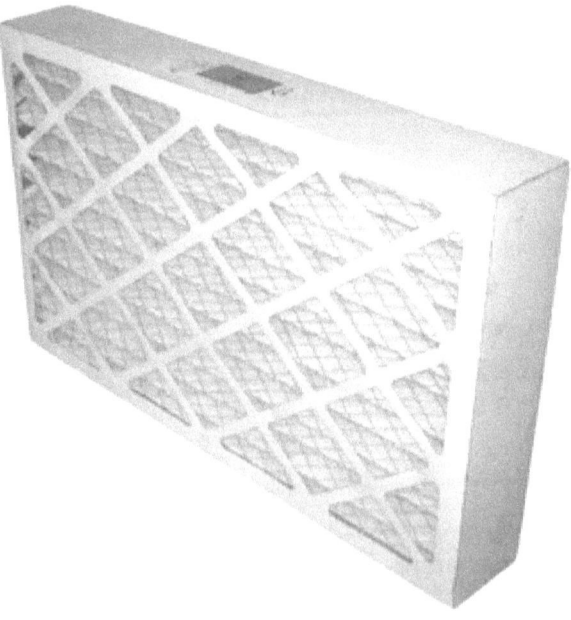

2. After that, we proceed with the measurement of the size of the filter needed for the mask and cut the shape: it should be about 12 cm tall and 18-19 cm wide.

It is important to remember that the measures shown here are indicative, the size of the mask depends on the size of the face.

3. Remove the rhombus pattern layer from the filter and throw it away

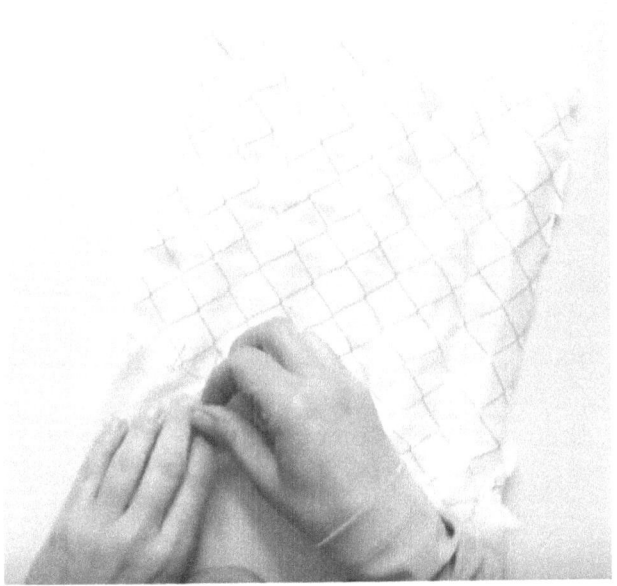

4. Paste one of the two shapes of fabric to solidify it and to "seal it" further.

5. The next step is to put the right side of the filter (the one with the metallic part) on the shape that has been strengthen in the point before.

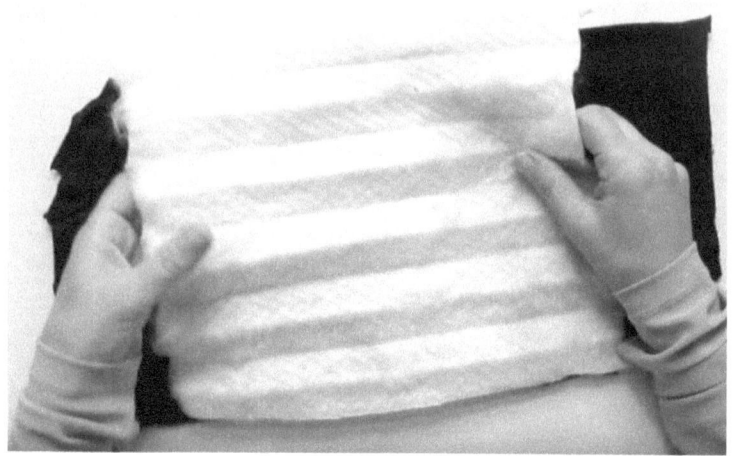

6. Put the last layer of fabric on the filter layer and fix them together. Stitch on two opposite sides which will become the top and the bottom.

7. Slide the ends of an elastic band or the fine strip of cloth into each corner and pin it by forming a loop inside the mask. Sew. Do the same on the opposite edge, making sure to leave a 6 cm slit so that you can turn the mask over.

8. Iron and notch (only) the angles, taking care not to cut the elastics.

9. Turn over and bring out the edges with a pen tip. Iron. Close the slit by sewing by hand with slip stitches.

10. Form three flat folds in the middle of the mask: fold the fabric over 1 cm (well parallel to the top and bottom) and by folding this fold down. Repeat twice. Iron.

11. Stitch these folds as close as possible to the edge. We have just created a new face mask version, but with a stronger filter.

Chapter Seven

For Those Who Do Not Have A Sewing Machine

Faced with the shortage of stocks of protective medical masks, we are all concerned by the spread of the Coronavirus virus. Also, in disarray faced with the shortage of stocks of medical masks when doubts about our health arise, all the more so when we live with frail, elderly, or young people. For lack of better, this free tutorial of a protective mask in the washable fabric or even paper towel may be useful to you. Unlike the first, this protective mask does not replace a normal mask. Its purpose is to prevent the spread in the air and the environment of saliva particles, potentially contaminated by the virus.

Necessary materials:

- A sheet of paper towel.

- ⬚ Elastics.

- ⬚ A stapler.

You can get all the materials at Amazon or Alibaba website.

The Steps To Follow:

1. Wash your hands and decontaminate them with hydroalcoholic gel.

2. Unfold the paper towel and fold it into an accordion together with the filter.

3. Place a rubber band at each end and staple them

Only use the face mask once, and for no more than 3 to 4 hours before replacing with a new mask.

Below are the pictures representation of the recipe:

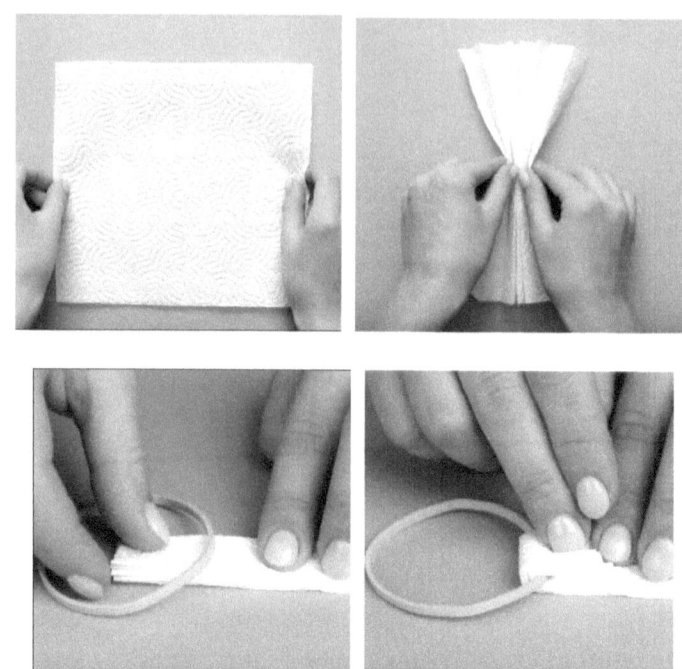

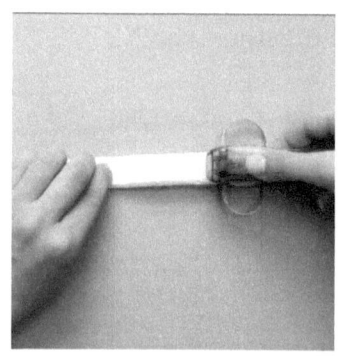

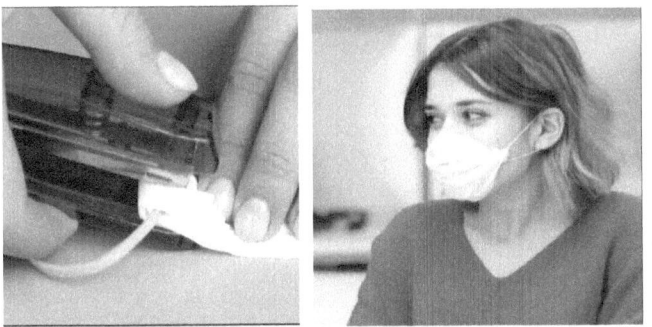

IMPORTANT: be sure to change this protective mask as soon as it becomes wet.

Conclusion

With masks sold out during the coronavirus outbreak, many people will have to make mask with what some scientists have called "the last resort": the DIY mask.

Data shows that DIY and homemade masks are effective at capturing viruses. But if forced to make our own mask, what material is best suited to make a mask? As the coronavirus spread around China, citizens reported making masks with tissue paper, kitchen towels, cotton clothing fabrics, and even oranges!

Now that we have outlined details on the types of surgical masks, how surgical masks are made and challenge to companies trying to break into the field, we hope this will enable you to source more effectively. If the problem is filtration effectiveness, would the masks work better if we doubled up with two layers of fabric? The scientists tested virus-size particles against double-layered versions of the dishtowel, pillowcase, and 100% cotton shirt fabrics.

Whatever you choose to use, make sure that you do not share it with anybody else. After getting overused, damaged, or soiled put it inside a plastic bag and throw it into the trash bin.